# How I Co
# High Cholesterol
# Through
# Diet and Exercise

## Liz  Broomfield

ISBN: 1508747776

ISBN-13: 978-1508747772

DEDICATION

To Matthew

# CONTENTS

ACKNOWLEDGEMENTS ......................................7

INTRODUCTION: MY STORY ...............................9

MEDICAL WARNINGS .......................................13

OTHER SOURCES OF HELP ...............................17

THE BASICS ....................................................19

MY DIET GUIDELINES ......................................27

MY EXERCISE GUIDELINES...............................33

FOODS I CAN EAT ...........................................37

FOODS I CAN'T EAT .........................................51

EATING OUT ...................................................55

THE END GAME: WHAT IT'S ALL ABOUT ..........63

RECIPES ..........................................................69

ABOUT THE AUTHOR ......................................73

ABOUT MY BOOKS ..........................................75

# ACKNOWLEDGEMENTS

This booklet is dedicated to Matthew and my friends, who have put up with all the oats, and the fussiness when eating out – thank you for your support and understanding!

Particular thanks to all my beta readers, especially Gill for proofreading and Pauline for being the first to use it

# INTRODUCTION: MY STORY

In May 2010 I had a regular blood test I need because I'm on blood pressure medication, which showed a raised cholesterol level of 7.1 (274 in the US*). Although the guidelines on what constituted "high" cholesterol had changed, this was seen as A Bad Thing by my doctor. They wanted to put me on Statins immediately. However, I wasn't yet 40, and I didn't really want to be on another lot of drugs for the rest of my life. I had also heard a few reports about side-effects of Statins that I wanted to avoid if I could.

So I asked my doctor if I could have a year to work on my cholesterol levels naturally. At that point, all I knew was that fat was "bad" for cholesterol, and I was aware that, although I generally ate healthily, and was fit and active, there was a fair amount of chocolate, biscuits and cake in my diet.

I asked for advice from the doctor and was given a single sheet of general advice for all population groups. As I don't eat much ghee or coconut oil, this was great in general but not brilliant for me, specifically. I did end up having an appointment to discuss my diet with the nurse, but on the whole I did this on my own.

In August 2010, my reading was down to 6.4 (247) with a fair amount of "good" cholesterol (see below for all about that). So I was allowed to stay off the Statins. Phew! By May 2011 it was 6.1 (235), and in March 2012 it got down to 5.1 (196) – the "safe" level is 5 (200), so I was well and truly there. My blood pressure has also come down, so now I'm on just half the dose of my low-dose medication that I started on.

How did I do this? I put myself on what seemed to be quite a harsh diet regime, and upped my exercise. I'm going to explain more about this as you read this short book – with lots of specific things that helped me, and some hints about eating out and treats.

I would like to save you from bursting into tears in Tesco's when you find that dark chocolate DOES have fat in it … and to help a few more people navigate the possibilities of controlling cholesterol levels naturally and keeping off the pills.

So in this booklet, I'm going to:

Explain the medical bits and show you where you can find more information

Talk about my "rules" and how they are applied in practice

Tell you about some things you'll be surprised you can eat, and some you'll be surprised you can't

Have a quick word about places you can eat out without undermining your diet

Go through some exercise tips

Please read the medical warnings that come next – then I hope you find this information useful!

# MEDICAL WARNINGS

I am not your doctor. Anything you choose to do in response to this booklet is your own responsibility. Please see your doctor if you have any concerns about your health at all.

This booklet is aimed at people who have slightly raised cholesterol levels and, with the agreement of their doctor, are trying to reduce them naturally.

There are many theories about ways to treat high cholesterol. Statins and other drugs are one way to do this. If you have dangerously high cholesterol and other factors that affect your cardiovascular health, there is always the option of going on the pills, adjusting your diet anyway, then seeing if your cholesterol levels improve further.

Once you have tweaked your diet in the ways I suggest, it's worth talking to your practice nurse or dietician about your diet, bringing in a diet sheet, to check through it and make sure you're making healthy choices. As you'll read, I did this, and it was very useful.

Please: if you have very high cholesterol or have been prescribed drugs, don't just ignore the doctor's advice. Talk to your doctor, try out some of my ideas, and see how it goes, while on your drugs, if you need them.

Other people suggest cutting down carbs and other ways to reduce cholesterol. All I can say is that this way of approaching things has worked for me. It's also worked for a couple of my friends: so it's worth a try. It's a healthy way of eating, anyway, and that's got to be good!

IF YOU ARE TRYING TO BECOME PREGNANT – some recent research has shown that a diet rich in low fat dairy products may inhibit your chances of getting pregnant. Take your doctor's advice, particularly if you are trying to conceive.

Please note that the information in this booklet was written primarily for a UK audience. I include details of the different measures of cholesterol used in different parts of the world, and I am going to talk about some places to eat out which may not exist or have different menus in your region. However, most of the basic information is the same wherever you are, so please do read on, but be aware of this.

# OTHER SOURCES OF HELP

I would like to say thank you to the charity, HEART UK, for their support of my project. They took the time to read this book, and HEART UK's dietician, Linda Main, was kind enough to provide me with this quotation, which I'm permitted to use in this book and the promotional materials around it:

"Liz provides some practical common-sense ideas and advice which she has tried and tested to lower and maintain healthy cholesterol levels. Her results demonstrate how a healthy balanced diet, low in saturated fat and high in wholegrain, fruits and vegetables and containing some cholesterol busting foods such as oats and nuts can be a central part of achieving this."

HEART UK can be found online at www.heartuk.org.uk and they have lots of information about how to deal with high cholesterol.

# THE BASICS: WHAT IS HIGH CHOLESTEROL AND WHAT ARE THE DIFFERENT TYPES OF FAT?

**What is high cholesterol?**

Cholesterol is a fatty substance, or "lipid" which is made by the liver and can be found in some foods. If you have too much cholesterol in your blood, it can affect your health, by increasing your risk of serious health conditions including coronary diseases such as angina, strokes and heart attacks.

Cholesterol is carried around the body by two kinds of protein:

Low-density lipoprotein (LDL or "bad" cholesterol) – this carries cholesterol from your liver to where it's needed. Too much to carry? It dumps it in your arteries, where it builds up on the walls

High-density lipoprotein (HDL or "good" cholesterol) – this one carries cholesterol back from the cells into the liver, where it is broken down or passed out of the body in the waste.

## Why is high cholesterol bad?

There is a lot of evidence that high cholesterol can increase the risk of narrowing of the arteries, heart attack and stroke (including mini-stroke), as well as blood clots.

All this is because of that depositing of the excess cholesterol in the arteries, restricting the flow of blood to your heart, brain, etc.

## What are the causes of high cholesterol?

The main factors that contribute to high cholesterol are:

- An unhealthy diet full of dietary cholesterol (cholesterol actually present in foods, although the medical sector seems to change how bad they think this is to consume!) and particularly saturated fat
- Smoking – there's a chemical in cigarettes which stops HDL from carrying the LDL away to the liver
- Family history. The inherited condition, familial hypercholesterolaemia can cause really high cholesterol, even in people who eat healthily.

Your risk of having a cardiovascular problem if you have high cholesterol is increased if you …

- Have diabetes or high blood pressure
- Have a family history of stroke or heart disease

## How do I find out more?

It's worth having a full cholesterol test (make sure they measure HDL and LDL as well as the total) and also a Cardiovascular Risk Assessment, which is something your GP surgery should offer. This will pick up your total risk of a cardiovascular health issue like a heart attack or a stroke. If your risk is reasonably low, and the doctor says it's OK, go on to try out the hints and tips in this booklet. If your risk is high, do what the doctor says about pills or whatever, then try these tips anyway.

For more information on high cholesterol, try the NHS website – for example their High Cholesterol pages.

**Measuring cholesterol**
As I discovered when trying to find out more information about my own condition, they measure things totally differently in the UK and US!

The UK (and Canada) measure cholesterol levels in units of millimoles per litre (mmol/L), whereas the US uses milligrams per decilitre (mg/DL).

To convert between the two, you use a factor of 38.6598 to multiply (UK to US) or divide (US to UK). I've put both in the "my story" section above to make it easier. I found a handy converter online.

Interestingly, this makes the "safe" levels slightly different in the UK and US. The target is 5 in the UK but 200 in the US, which equates to 5.18.

Before starting using the tips in this booklet, you need to know your types of fat. There are four:

## Saturated fat
The baddy! This is the one that helps raise your cholesterol. Actually, we don't really know why. It has something to do with "belly fat", and I have to say that when I went on this diet, my tummy did get a bit thinner (the rest of me didn't lose weight: this is not particularly a weight loss diet if you have a reasonable diet and weight already. You might do if you have some very unhealthy eating habits).

You find saturated fat in animal products, including

Red meat, especially fatty cuts

Meat products, like sausages, pies, etc.

Butter, lard, ghee and cheese (especially hard cheese), cream and ice cream

Snacks and some sweets

Cakes, biscuits and pastries

Oh no! I hear you cry. But don't fear: there are lots of alternatives! It's taken me a while to find them, so I'll save you time and upset by telling you about them later.

## Trans fats

Trans fats are another kind of fat that can raise cholesterol levels in the blood. Trans fats are found in animal products too, and in foods containing hydrogenated vegetable oil. Although there has been some fuss about these recently, in the UK we don't actually eat a lot of these. Most supermarkets have removed them from their own brand products.

Hydrogenated vegetable oil has to be listed on the ingredients of products. So keep an eye out and just to be on the safe side, avoid these.

## Polyunsaturated fats

Hooray – now we're on to the good ones!

Polyunsaturated fats tend to lower both "bad" LDL cholesterol and "good" HDL cholesterol. They include safflower oil, sunflower oil and corn oil.

## Monounsaturated fats

The good guys. These ones tend to lower the bad LDL cholesterol and leave your good, HDL, cholesterol levels alone. They include canola oil and olive oil.

In general, saturated fats are solid at room temperature (think blocks of lard sitting in your arteries!) and unsaturated fats are liquid – oils.

## You do need fat, though!

Don't cut out all fat! The trick is to get a good balance where you're eating enough monounsaturated and polyunsaturated fats in order to give you the essential fatty acids you need to keep your body functioning. Fat is needed to help your cell membranes maintain themselves, and to keep things running smoothly.

Essential fatty acids

You can find essential fatty acids, including omega-3 and omega-6 in vegetable oils, fish, grains, seeds and vegetables.

You may find you need to take a supplement when you reduce the fat in your diet. My skin and hair went a bit dry and scaly (nice!)

so I added in a Cod Liver Oil capsule once a day and felt a lot better and less itchy.

Get used to seeking out this information on the back of food packets. It should all be there (note: sometimes it's printed REALLY small. I'm 40, I can't read small print very well. Still read it).

Right, now we know about the kinds of fat, let's look at how it all works in practice.

# MY DIET GUIDELINES

There really was not much help when I started looking into this. That's why I'm putting all this information together for you now! So, in this section, I'm going to tell you all about the rules that have helped me lower my cholesterol.

They're pretty simple, and should be easy to follow – I've used them fairly rigorously and they worked for me, and you'll find that you get used to checking the packaging on food or information on menus and identifying the details you need – and what you can eat – quickly and easily after a little bit of practice.

**Maximum 1% saturated fat**

This is my basic rule. I look at the packet, or the guidelines in the nutritional information pack provided by the café or restaurant (see below). 1% saturated fat means 1g per 100g. Be careful when looking at the information panel. Often they show you fat, etc., per bar, or per serving. That's fine for later: for now, find the amount per 100g.

1% = 1g per 100g

**Maximum 5g saturated fat per meal**

Help! Maths! I'm not very good at maths, but this is OK to work out, because the nutritional information will tell you how much "stuff" there is in your food per portion.

If you look at the front of your food packet and it says it weighs less than 100g, and you already know it contains less than 1% saturated fat, you're fine. No maths!

Items that weigh more than 100g may have more fat than you want. Maths time! It's not that hard, though.

Say your lasagne has 1% saturated fat. Hooray! But look, it weighs 700g. 1% sat fat = 1g per 100g. Multiply your 1g by 7 and you get … 7g. That's a bit much. Put it down. Or buy it and only eat half of it (see the end section, you'll probably find it a bit greasy anyway).

## Nasty surprises

Just looking at the nutritional labels can give you some nasty surprises. "Oh, I'm sure I can have DARK chocolate," I said to myself. Oh. So it's worth checking what you can and can't have. I went round the supermarket making a big list when I went on this diet, then it was easier to know which of my favourites I could still have. Also: note that there are some nice surprises, too. In a few chapters' time, I'll share some of those with you.

## Exceptions and treats

Some things are worth going over that 1% rule (however, I wouldn't go over the 5g rule). There are a few categories here:

- The balance between unsaturated and saturated fats. If something has "too much" saturated fat but whopping great gobbets of unsaturated fat (I'm thinking olive oil and avocados here) then go for it. I don't have a standard rule here, but if something has more than 10 times the unsaturated fat than the saturated, I'll still eat it

- Some things you can't live without. For me, it's cheese and chocolate (I used to be allergic to both of these: was my body trying to tell me something?). I have yet to find a cheese with less than 1% saturated fat. I have found two that I will eat: Minicol (which has Benecol, which MAY lower cholesterol in it) and Wyke Farms SuperLight Cheese (more on that later, but 1.5% saturated fat is AMAZING for a cheddar – check even the "low fat" varieties and you'll see what I mean). With chocolate, I go for the darkest, highest quality chocolate I can find, and have ONE PIECE once a week. Amazingly (and those who knew me in the great Giving Up Chocolate For A Month trauma back in the day will be truly amazed), I can cope with this. It is actually nicer than cramming in mouthfuls of cheap milk chocolate.

- Butter / spreads / mayonnaise –
  pretty well all butter and spread has
  "too much" fat but look at those
  balances and go for the most "good"
  fat vs. least "bad" fat combo. I use
  the Flora extra light – olive oil
  spread is OK, too, but watch out for
  the ones that aren't made just out of
  olive oil but have added ingredients.
  And don't go mad with them – a thin
  spread or try just leaving it out
  altogether. Cook with other
  ingredients, too (like olive oil) rather
  than slathering fat into recipes. As
  for mayonnaise, the WeightWatchers
  varieties are low fat, or make your
  own salad dressing with olive oil and
  balsamic vinegar, etc.

# MY EXERCISE GUIDELINES

The research says that exercise raises good cholesterol (the HDL stuff that clears out the arteries and pops it back into the liver for processing and eliminating). My research on myself seems to back that up – not only did my total go down, but the proportion made up of good cholesterol went up.

I already went running 3 times a week, but I increased the time I spend exercising and I try to make sure I get some vigorous exercise every day.

The NHS / Government recommend 30 minutes of brisk exercise, 5 times a week. They define this as exercise that gets you out of breath and sweating (but not crawling around gasping).

Of course, talk to your doctor before embarking upon an exercise programme, especially if you have other health issues, don't normally take much exercise, etc.

If you do already exercise, break it up a bit. You might be super fit in your normal exercise routine and have trouble getting your heart pounding and working up a sweat. I have trouble getting that walking, unless I go really fast or up and down hills. So that's what I do. I also added a lot of cross-training and weights to my exercise routine.

You don't need to join a gym – you can go walking, go for a run, do press-ups in the park or stretches on a bench. Bicep curls with cans of baked beans … the opportunities are endless.

A typical week for me:

Monday – rest day but a brisk walk towards my husband's office to meet him walking home

Tuesday – 1 hour gym session. 30 mins on the cross-trainer or bike, 30 minutes with the weights

Wednesday – 1 hour on the exercise bike, having a read! But still working hard and sweating

Thursday – same as Monday or Tuesday, or a 45 minute run

Friday – same as Tuesday or Wednesday

Saturday – general running around, in town, etc.

Sunday – an hour's run outdoors

I try for 4-5 hours of exercise a week. It keeps me happy and toned and gives me an appetite, too.

If you hate gyms, the walking will do it – or Zumba classes, or tennis … you'll find it's easier to do this if it's to improve your health as well as lose weight or because you "should".

# FOODS I CAN EAT

Getting right down to the nitty-gritty, here are the foods around which I base my diet:

WHOLE GRAINS

These keep you full for longer, don't mess with your blood sugar levels and the fibre in them can help reduce your cholesterol too! The blood sugar thing means you're less likely to crave sweet, fatty foods that aren't so good for you.

Examples:

Brown rice

Brown pasta (I actually prefer the flavour of these – mix them with white at first if you think they'll taste like cardboard)

Shreddies or the like for breakfast

Wholegrain bread

OATS

Yes, I know oats are a wholegrain. But they're also a bit of a miracle food. They, along with apples and other fruits and veg, are a source of soluble fibre. And soluble fibre acts a bit like that stuff you pour down your drains, scouring out the cholesterol build-up from your body and popping it in the good old liver for disposal. I am pretty sure that oats and running are what have sorted my cholesterol levels out. Note: oats do have some fat in them (I don't know where that is, but it's there) but they are recommended for their soluble fibre, so that's fine.

Here's how I use my lovely oats:

At breakfast time. One of the things you always hear about cholesterol lowering diets is porridge. So I tried it. Oh, how I cried over my porridge. Ugh, ugh, ugh. Turns out

I don't like hot milk. On occasion, I'll have a bowl of oats with cold milk. This is NOT cold porridge, it's just like cereal. But I always have a bag of oats around, and I always add a couple of tablespoonfuls to my cereal of a morning. If you want muesli, making it yourself with a base of oats will guarantee you can control what's in it

In sauces, soups and other cooking. I have a bag of oat bran at the ready. Sprinkle a couple of spoonfuls in at the beginning of the cooking process, and it absorbs in, you can't see it, your sauce is prevented from going watery, and you've got your soluble fibre without even thinking about it.

At pudding time. Fat free yoghurt, oats and honey. Yum!

MEAT

I do have to be careful with meat as it can contain fats. But if you go for very lean cuts, take the skin off chicken, eat lots of turkey, then you're fine. I have a little bit of thinly sliced ham sometimes, a fair bit of chicken … and you can get bacon without the fat on which is OK. I'm lucky in that I don't eat much meat anyway. Oh, the great one …

Ostrich burgers! Ostrich has almost no saturated fat. Go to your local farmers' market and I bet there's an ostrich burger stall. Watch what they fry them in, but hooray – a proper red meat burger!

I hear that kangaroo is the same … but wild boar isn't, and a stallholder at a Christmas Market did try to convince me it was, so watch out there.

## MEAT SUBSTITUTES

Quorn is my friend. Luckily, I really like quorn. It's low fat and high protein and comes in all sorts of forms, including slices to put in your sandwiches, lovely sausages, and mince and chunks for cooking with. Make Quorn your friend, too!

## FISH

Oily fish are good for you (unless you're pregnant or breast-feeding, in which case you need to keep an eye on mercury). If you like sardines-in-a-tin, all to the good, but any fish is better than none. Oh, and eat the skin on this, as that's where those omega fatty acids live that are so good for you.

## BEANS, PULSES, VEGETABLES

You are looking to get some soluble fibre into you to help the oats sweep away those nasty lipids. So lots of things like chickpeas and other beans as well as lots of veg will fill you up nicely. Dried fruit is fine, too, but I tend to steer clear of fruit and nut mixes, as nuts vary in their goodness and fat levels.

## NUTS AND SEEDS

Nuts and seeds can be a bit iffy. Peanuts are full of fat – but so are other nuts that are good for you. As a general rule, I go for …

Walnuts – these are the "best" nut for us cholesterol-lowerers

Almonds – also good

Linseeds – as well as their oil, these are good whole. Sprinkle them on your morning cereal!

## OILS

Olive oil is good and the other good ones are linseed and safflower. We cook with a linseed oil and you can get avocado oil, too. Have a look at what your supermarket offers and try to get the proportion of saturated to unsaturated fats as heavily biased towards the unsaturated as you can. They can differ in taste, so do try a few!

## SKIMMED MILK

You will learn to embrace the bluish purity of skimmed milk. It took me a few goes, but I genuinely like it now. And it actually has more calcium and protein than even semi-skimmed (presumably because there's nothing else in it). Note that in cafes, if you ask for skimmed milk they will ALMOST ALWAYS say, brightly, "Semi skimmed!". But sometimes they won't and they do have skimmed. Hooray!

As well as skimmed milk, you could try naturally low fat soya milk or oat milk – that's quite nice and will give you that soluble fibre, but it is pretty expensive.

If you want to get soya milk into your coffee without that vile blobbiness, by the way, pour it into a spoon first. I don't know why this works, but it does.

## PUDDINGS AND CAKES AND SWEETS

I have given up trying to keep the sugar levels right down as well. Yes, you shouldn't go mad, but you can't have no treats, and unless you're diabetic or pre-diabetic, and as long as you're sensible, have a few bits and pieces that you can have.

Yoghurt – there's loads of fat free yoghurt around. If, like me, you don't get on with the pro-biotic ones, then Weightwatchers do some good ones. Fat free yoghurt with some honey and fruit – yum!

Fruit – always good and you can combine it with the jolly things in this list too

Low fat ice cream – all the supermarkets do a non-dairy ice cream like substance. No, it's not vanilla, but look at the fat in that … and it does very well once you've got over the pain of giving up real ice cream

Meringues – only made with egg whites and sugar. In fact, they're very easy to make yourself, as long as you've got an electric whisk. They feel really, really treat-y and are quite cheap, too

Hard boiled and jelly sweets are generally OK, toffees and fudge not. Most carry nutritional information, but some don't – be aware.

IN GENERAL

I find that vegan products are often good, as they won't have animal fats in them. Look at the labels. You'll see that this is a general healthy diet, with some sweets and puddings that your dieting friends would avoid. Not too bad, really …

You will end up cooking from scratch more, and planning meals and snacks more. But is that really a bad thing?

What I would repeat, is go around the supermarket and look at the labels in a whole section at a time. Look at your favourites, see if you can still have them. If not, is there an alternative? Note it down, then you've got a list for when it gets all overwhelming later on.

## A note about the cholesterol reducing products

There are products which say they contain cholesterol reducing chemicals. Have a look at the dose required. One of the cheeses I eat, well, I would blanch at the amount that makes up a portion and I like my cheese. They are also pretty expensive. If you don't eat much spread anyway, I personally feel that a bit of the lowest fat spread you can find is OK.

There are also natural products, usually called "plant sterols", that claim to help. I tried these, and they didn't do anything for me. They're also quite expensive. What I suggest here is, get your levels measured, try the things for a few months, keeping the rest of your diet the same as before, and get tested again. If they make a difference: great.

## Surprising foods I can eat

I have caused surprise when spotted eating certain foods – and these are the ones we tend to gleefully share when we find out about them. I think sometimes people assume that anyone with a food issue needs gluten free, and I do have to explain that quite often, but these are foods you maybe didn't think you could have … but you can!

Muffins from Starbucks – hooray for Starbucks, as we'll discuss in the Eating Out section. Actually, quite a lot of cafes and restaurants are now much better at providing nutritional information. I don't know what Starbucks Skinny Muffins are made out of, and they are quite high-calorie and high-sugar treats, but, oh, it's nice to just sit down and eat a blooming CAKE once in a while, without having to make it myself!

Cakes – home-made cakes are more than possible. Have a Google. The best way to replace the fat seems to be with apple sauce or other fruits. There's a recipe at the back of this book for a lovely Plum cake. And commercially, you can find the odd one. The Mrs Crimble's brand, usually found in the "Free From" or special diets section of the supermarket, does an Apple Cake which is very low fat and not gluten-free, although it's in that section.

Another cake-like treat is Tea Bread or Barra Brith. Because it's a raisiny bread rather than a cake, it's made of bread ingredients and low fat. Hooray! If you're in Birmingham, both branches of Urban Coffee Company stock it. And also have a look at Hot Cross Buns and tea cakes – both fine when not in the "Finest" / "Extra special" supermarket ranges and not, of course, slathered in butter. Hot cross buns can be bought all year round and are great to pop in your bag for emergency consumption.

Biscuits – sponge fingers, amaretti biscuits. Sponge fingers aren't just for trifles, but they are OK as a biscuit. Amaretti biscuits are made of ground up almond stones and not much else. Oh, my joy when I discovered I could eat them! I actually jumped up and down in the office where I then worked!

Pizza – Well done, Pizza Express, who do a Leggera range of pizzas that have a hole in the middle for salad, and a low-fat base, coming in at 5g or so of saturated fat per pizza. Fine for a treat and so nice to be able to eat out somewhere other people like to go, too. You can also make your own pizzas with low-fat cheese and a low fat base and any toppings you fancy.

Curry – it is possible to ask for your curry to be made with no oil at your local curry house. Also, a lot of the ready meals now have pretty low fat, and onion bhajis etc. and even naans are available in the supermarket. Watch out for the sugar (see below), but it's just nice to have "normal" food every now and then.

Chinese – again, check out fat levels in different ready meals and ingredients and you may be pleasantly surprised. Sweet and sour sauce is fine, as long as it's not covering deep-fried anything, and prawns are also fine these days, even though they do contain some cholesterol themselves.

Cheese – three cheers for Wyke Farms Super Light Somerset cheddar. It tastes like real cheese, but has 1.5% saturated fat – which is amazing. The reason they make it is that a member of the farmer's family was diagnosed with high cholesterol – so they made a cheese for him! It's available in Asda and the Coop, and you can order it online from Wyke Farms' website. There is another cheese called Minicol, which has higher fat but contains a cholesterol-lowering ingredient. However, as I have mentioned, you need to eat a heck of a lot of it to get the cholesterol-lowering portion. It does melt well, and it is available in Sainsbury's, so worth a look.

Eggs – guidelines change massively on these. I can't say I actually LIKE eggs, although I know they're full of protein – so I tend to just eat the whites in meringues. They do contain cholesterol, but medical science now seems to say that eating cholesterol isn't as bad as manufacturing it yourself. The NHS website doesn't have any guidelines on this. So, you can eat them, but don't go mad.

## A note on low-fat ready meals, etc.

You may be surprised to know that, to make up for the fat and the tastiness that goes with it, ready meals and other low-fat foods are stuffed full of sugar. This is true, but what's also true is that a terribly worthy diet stuffed full of lentils and prunes will drive you mad and send you on a path towards bingeing on fatty foods and making yourself feel horrible.

I say that as long as you don't have them all the time, and maybe get your blood glucose levels checked once a year or so, it's fine to indulge in these once in a while. Don't make yourself miserable for the sake of it.

# FOODS I CAN'T EAT

This is the giving up section. But I'm going to try to be positive here. It's not all bad. I'll try to give you an alternative for each one …

Red meat – that protein is so often associated with saturated fat. But look at the labels. Choose very good steak when it's on special offer. Go to the farmers' market and pick up a tray of ostrich burgers, freeze them, and have a lovely burger whenever you want.

Cheese – but there are alternatives (see "Surprising foods I can eat" above)

Crisps – but again, there are alternatives. Pretzels – oh, the joy. And a lot of baked and other magical crisps. You do not actually have to give up crisps

Biscuits and cakes – yes, these are full of sat fat. Actually, they look and smell a bit vile once you've avoided them for a while (I PROMISE!). You can find recipes for making all sorts of lovelies that rely on egg substitute or apple sauce and other fruits to make them moist and stick together. So you might end up doing more baking, but I bet the end result is nicer and free from additives!

Chocolate – this was the hardest one for me. But, honestly, a small bit of good chocolate once a week does satisfy me now. I promise. And anyone who knows me knows that is odd.

Shop-bought sandwiches – this is a monumental pain, actually. Look for the salmon and cucumber ones, and get more creative with your packed lunches. That's all I can say there.

Meals out – this is really hard and gets its own section in a chapter or so. But it is

possible, and places are getting better a)
with giving nutritional information and b)
with understanding about "odd" diets.


### Surprising foods I can't eat

Oatcakes – oats, yes. Oatcakes appear to be
made of lard. This annoys me, but it's
unfortunately true.

Sweets – watch out – some of them have
loads of fat in them. Some seem to have it to
stop them sticking together, some to make a
hard shell, I assume (Skittles, I'm looking at
you here). Look at the nutritional content
and you'll be fine.

Different varieties of the same product.
Today I was looking at some individual
portions of banana bread and a loaf. The
individuals claimed 0.8% fat, the loaf, 1.5%.
I left them on the shelf.

Sports nutrition drinks and supplements – if
you use the gym a lot you will have these
waved in front of you. But they mostly
contain a fair bit of saturated fat. It does lead
to an interesting conversation about your
funny diet, though!

"Just for a treat"

This annoys me a bit. I don't really want to eat fatty treats, to be honest. I've been avoiding fatty foods for a number of years now, and I really don't like the taste – or smell – of them. Biscuits smell like a chip shop to me, and doughnuts like hell on earth. So don't offer me – or us – a treat and say "just this once", if you're reading this in support of a friend trying the diet. Oh – fatty foods also upset my stomach. This is common.

# EATING OUT (OR, BEWARE THE SIDE DISH)

Ah: the difficult one. Eating out. I love my friend who's on Weightwatchers (she's lost 8 stone and kept it off so she must be doing something right). When we go out in a group, she and I can be awkward together! Hooray! Otherwise, it can be a monumental pain.

Here's what I've found out.

## Snacks

For a lunchtime snack, you are going to get really sick and tired of the jacket potato (no butter) with baked beans (no cheese). Oh, I said no cheese, sorry. Or butter. But that is often on any café or pub menu, and it does fill you up and give you some protein, fibre and carbs. I did get VERY excited the other day when I had a choice of two jacket potato fillings. It was a shame the salad came laced with mayonnaise, but you can't have everything!

Teacakes are often on offer in cafes and are a good option, without the butter. And we've already talked about muffins in Starbucks. Starbucks and Costa have full nutritional information packs available behind the counter. You have to ask (see "dealing with eating establishments" below) and you will probably find that only one or two foods are available, but it's helpful to be able to see what's available and possible.

At a pinch, I'll have a hummus sandwich or wrap, or falafels – vegetarian is safe, hummus and falafels are full of unsaturated fats and fibre … so look for those options.

For pub food, Wetherspoons pubs have full nutritional information readily available, and do some vege chillies, etc., which are more than possible with the odd tweak to remove the crisps. They seem to be able to remove or not add sour cream and the like, too. Lots of pub meals are ready-prepared, but if you're in less of a chain pub, ask the kitchen if they can change things slightly. You can do it!

There are some other, independent food providers who can be excellent. I want to make a special mention of Kuskus Foods here (www.kuskusfoods.co.uk/). Moe has the inherited version of very high cholesterol, so pretty well everything he cooks is suitable for a cholesterol-beating diet. Kuskus has stalls at farmers' markets throughout the Midlands, and it's well worth stocking up on falafels and other delicacies (tell him I sent you!).

## Main meals

I have to admit that I have ended up limiting my eating out to a few chain restaurants that I know I can eat at. It's a shame, but it's such a palaver otherwise. Here are my favourites:

Sushi! Nowadays, there is often an all you can eat sushi bar in your local town or city. Birmingham has Woktastic www.woktastic.co.uk , which offers good value and is actually suitable for

vegetarians, gluten free and fat free folks.
The trick is to just go for the standard items
– rolls and the blocks of rice with fish laid
on top. No fat there, and some fish – often
oily – too. As long as you avoid the deep
fried items, you can eat and eat and eat!

Wagamama (www.wagamama.co.uk) – as
long as you avoid the fattier meats,
Wagamama offers choice for the fat free
diner. Again, they provide nutritional
information upon request. I find the clear
soups with wholemeal noodles and
vegetable sauces are great – again, avoid the
deep-fried options.

Pizza Express (www.pizzaexpress.com) – as
previously mentioned, they do a Leggera
range of pizzas which we can eat. I now eat
much more at PE than I ever did before!

Las Iguanas (www.iguanas.co.uk) – a chain
of South American themed restaurants:
you'd think it'd all be tortillas and cheese,
but first of all, they have a range of low fat
dishes – I can usually get a choice of two or
three mains, and secondly they are willing to
tweak dishes for you, so, for example, they
will do you their goat's cheese salad without

the goat's cheese. And they don't just pick it out of the salad, either!

## Restaurants in the US

My America correspondent reports that Chipotle (www.chipotle.com) , Cosi (www.getcosi.com) and Panera (www.panerabread.com) all include full nutritional information on their websites – which is great. Do report back to me if you find good, possible meals at these places or any others.

## Hotels in the UK

I've found and stayed at two hotels in the UK which have both dealt admirably with my odd diet. Both also cater for gluten free, lactose free, vegetarian and vegan requirements.

Hillthwaite House Hotel in Windermere, the Lake District (www.hillthwaite.com) – they offer a half-board package with a fantastic five-course dinner every night – all catering to your dietary requirements.

Mountview Hotel and Restaurant in Nethy Bridge, near Aviemore, Scotland (www.mountviewhotel.co.uk) – I went there on a bird-watching holiday and they managed to cater for me full board, packed lunch included.

Please note: the above recommendations are personal recommendations. I have not been paid to include them in this book, and the experiences in them are my own.

## Dealing with eating establishments

It can be really tricky presenting yourself and your diet at a café or restaurant. I hate making a fuss, and of course I'm much quicker to complain about the meat on a friend's "veggie" pizza than to bring attention to myself. But I've worked out some ways to make the interaction easier.

Sometimes you have to ask what's in a meal, what it's been cooked in … what kind of milk it contains … whether the establishment has a set of nutritional information somewhere about the place. It's a bit embarrassing and it's important not to baffle your server with information or technical terms.

One of the big problems is that, for us, it's a "hidden" medical issue, in that I won't be made ill directly by the item (well, I feel unwell if I eat much fat now, but that's just being used to what I eat normally).

I have got it down to something like "I have a medical issue which means I cannot eat x. I am able to manage it without medication because I'm really careful, so it would be really great if you could check whether this has …. in it". I find mentioning "saturated fat" etc. really doesn't work very well – it has to be ridiculously clear: "I have a medical condition, this is what I cannot have".

I have found that 90% of the time this works really well. I have tried just "I can't eat fat" and get "oh, treat yourself", whether that is just because it's fat, I don't know, but introducing the medical issue right at the start seems to concentrate people and get them on-side.

In my case, it's not exactly the truth as I DON'T have high cholesterol because I control my diet – but, in my mind, I have a medical condition that means that if I eat much fat my cholesterol level will be raised. I have tried "an intolerance to fat" but that doesn't work as well.

If someone is particularly helpful about this, or just understanding, I make sure I thank and praise them, and let their manager know, if appropriate. I've filled in feedback forms in various cafes thanking and praising the staff. It all helps the next person.

One amusing thing you might find: if you ask for the nutritional information, sometimes they think you're a mystery shopper, testing them on their mastery of their workplace's more obscure features. Milk it! Only with skimmed milk though. And, of course, don't – but watch out for it!

# THE END GAME: WHAT IT'S ALL ABOUT

## Will I lose weight if I go on this diet?

This is not a weight-loss diet. In fact, I kind of recommend a load of sugary things. But if you have a diet that is particularly laden with red meat, chips and cakes, and no exercise, and you change to this diet, you may well end up losing weight.

If you're serious about losing weight, then

a) reduce calories in by controlling but not obsessing over your diet

b) increase calories out by taking more exercise

I do feel better on this diet than I used to, I have to say. And I have less fat in my body composition, so I do look a bit different!

What you will do, I think, is enjoy your food more: you'll almost inevitably be eating more home-cooked and fresher food, and that's always got to be good!

## Four years on and with normal cholesterol levels

When I first discovered I had "high" cholesterol and needed to take action to combat it, I got quite panicky and depressed. There were tears in the supermarket when I realised that, yes, dark chocolate does contain fat … That's why I've written this e-book, to help other people and make sure they don't have to struggle quite so hard.

It took me a while to work out what I could and couldn't eat. Obviously, different people like different foods, and you will need to take a look at the nutritional information on a few favourites and find substitutes, but hopefully the guidelines I've given will help a bit there.

Because it took me a while to work out what I could eat and how I could still eat a healthy, balanced diet, and because, frankly, it was a bit of a shock to have to do this in the first place, I did go a bit thin and grey-looking for a few weeks. And maybe a little obsessive. Some friends were concerned about me, and told me so. Others probably were, but didn't tell me.

I did take the important and useful step of keeping a food diary for a week or so and presenting it to the practice nurse at our doctor's surgery. She suggested a few tweaks: in my case, I wasn't eating quite enough protein, and she suggested some items I could add in to my lunches. This really helped me to work out a good and balanced diet that kept me well-nourished, healthy, and satisfied, while maintaining my cholesterol levels at an acceptable total.

I continued working out and running – in fact I added more workouts and variety into my exercise routine. As I have a desk-based job, I now make sure I get out and about, having some brisk exercise, for at least 30 minutes every day. And I've run two half-marathons since my diagnosis. While it is possible to do this and be undernourished and ill, it does show if you try to do that, and will take its toll in time. I'm my usual well-nourished and "solid" self, and feel that achieving these sporting milestones has demonstrated that the diet I'm on can support and enhance my training and running aims.

And those cholesterol levels? As I said at the beginning, I started off with total cholesterol of 7.1 (274 in the American measurement). In August 2010, my reading was down to 6.4 (247). By May 2011 it was 6.1 (235), and in March 2012 it got down to 5.1 (196) – the "safe" level is 5 (or 5.18/200 in the US), so I was well and truly there (and still is, at the time of creating this print book in March 2015).

I can't guarantee that you can get your cholesterol levels down in the same way that I did. A couple of my friends have managed it, but for a couple it didn't work. But I think it's worth trying, as long as you follow these steps:

- Talk to your doctor first

- If your levels are high enough to need statins, accept taking them and get the levels down while you're on them
- Tweak your diet and increase your exercise
- Consider taking a multivitamin and perhaps a cod liver oil capsule daily
- Book an appointment with a dietician or practice nurse trained in nutrition
- Have your levels tested regularly
- Talk to your doctor if you have any concerns

Good luck!

If you have any hotel or restaurant recommendations that could be added to a subsequent edition of this book, please get in touch at liz@libroediting.com to let me know.

Please do review this book on Amazon and/or your own book review blog or other place – it really does help to spread the word! Thank you.

# RECIPES

## Gill Rose's Plum Cake recipe

Ingredients:

450 g chopped plums

100 g white sugar

100 g brown sugar

1 egg white

250 g flour

1/2  teaspoon salt

1 heaped teaspoon baking powder

1 teaspoon vanilla essence

Half pint milk -- skimmed, sour or buttermilk

Topping:

100 grams white sugar

1  teaspoon cinnamon

Cream together sugars and egg. Add flour, salt, vanilla, baking powder, plums. Add milk to mix to a thick batter (more sloppy than a 'normal' sponge cake mixture). Pour into 10" cake tin. Top with mixture of sugar and cinnamon.

Bake at 325F for 50 minutes or until done (use a skewer to check).

I use skimmed milk, but you can make sour milk with a couple of tablespoons of white vinegar plus milk to equal one cup. Let stand while mixing rest of ingredients.

I've also made a smaller cake with half-quantities.

## Meringue recipe

This is a favourite of mine, and so easy! Meringues are a nice thing to take to parties or barbeques as they look indulgent (and are sugary) and almost everyone likes them.

Ingredients:

4 large egg whites

115g caster sugar

115g icing sugar


Preheat the oven to Gas Mark ¼ or 110 C.


Beat the egg whites in a clean metal or glass bowl until they stand up in peaks (please use an electric whisk for this – I did it with a balloon whisk once: not worth it).

Add the caster sugar a little at a time, as you continue beating. The mixture should start going all glossy. Yum!

At this stage, add coffee essence, strong black coffee, pieces of chopped strawberry, other flavourings and colourings, chopped walnuts – whatever you fancy!

Sift the icing sugar in a third at a time; fold it in to the mixture using a metal spoon.

Line baking sheets with parchment paper and dollop the mixture on (you can try to make nests or walnut whip shapes if you're feeling clever – I go for dollops). This should make about 16.

Bake in that cool oven for 1 hour 30 to 1 hour 45 – until the meringues are crisp and slightly golden. I then turn out the oven and leave them for a bit longer.

They will keep for about 2 weeks … yeah, right. I've never kept any that long.

# ABOUT THE AUTHOR

Liz Broomfield (the pen name of Liz Dexter) is an editor, transcriber, proofreader and localiser based in Birmingham, UK. She's passionate about sharing the lessons she's learned as someone who changed careers mid-life and is living a flexible and happy life doing work she loves, with time for the other things she loves in life.

Liz's books can be found on Amazon, Smashwords and Selz in print and all formats of e-book.

Visit Liz's book website at www.lizbroomfieldbooks.com

Visit Liz's business and Word tips website at www.libroediting.com

# ABOUT MY BOOKS

I write books that help self-employed people and people setting up and running small businesses to work out what to do first and what to do next. I write from my own experience, using lots of examples from my successful business life, and my books are all jargon-free, approachable and friendly. Most importantly, if you buy the book, you get the information that's promised. There's no requirement to buy a course or pay for additional materials. In fact, links and footnotes will take you to more FREE resources on my websites with screen shots and the latest updates. Find information, news and links to buy at www.lizbroomfieldbooks.com. Happy reading!

 "How I Survived my First Year of Full-Time Self-Employment: Going it Alone at 40" – all you need to know about setting up your new business and taking the plunge without too much risk or anxiety. Lots of personal stories and I share exactly how I did it – you don't need to buy any courses or additional resources to get the full value from this book.

"Running a Successful Business after the Start-up Phase or, Who are you Calling Mature?" – you've set up the business, you've been running for a couple of years, now it's time to refine your customer base, redress your work-life balance and think about add-ons like social media networking and blogging. This book tells you how and like its predecessor, shares real-life examples which show exactly how I've built a happy self-employed life for myself.

The business OMNIBUS "Your Guide to Starting and Building your Business" – why not save money on buying the above two books separately with this e-only guide to setting up and maintaining a successful and balanced business? I do like to provide value to my readers, and this includes the text of both books in full, put together in a special omnibus edition. It's downloadable in all of the different e-book formats or as a pdf to read on your computer or tablet.

"Quick Guide to Networking, Social Media and Social Capital" takes you through the benefits you can gain – and give – when you engage with people through face-to-face or social networking.

Printed in Great Britain
by Amazon